Making the Fast: How to Eat to Live During Ramadan

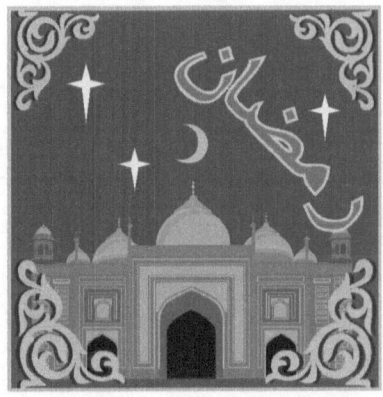

Raychelle Muhammad, B.S., CPT

DEDICATION

To members of the Believing family everywhere...

CONTENTS

DISCLAIMER

DISCLAIMER

This book provides information that is intended only to assist users in their efforts to complete the Ramadan fast. You are urged to seek the advice of a physician before beginning any fasting, diet, exercise, or weight loss/gain/management program. This book is intended for use only by healthy adult individuals. The book is not intended for use by minors, pregnant women, or individuals with any type of health condition. Such individuals are specifically warned to seek professional medical advice prior to initiating any form of fasting, diet, exercise, or weight loss/gain/management program.

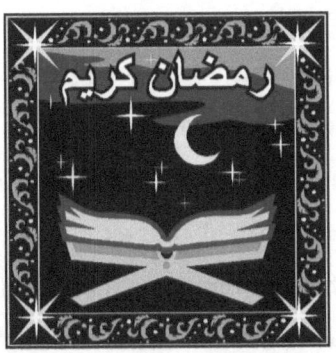

1 WHY WE FAST DURING RAMADAN

"FASTING takes away evil desires. Fasting takes from us filthy desires. Fasting takes from us the desire to do evil against self and our brothers and sisters. We are created of the material of goodness. Therefore, good belongs to us ... and it should not be hard for us to turn to our own selves in which we were created ... good." —**The Honorable Elijah Muhammad**

"The Honorable Elijah Muhammad taught us that fasting produces discipline. How? We know that we are creatures with desires and basic human needs: Food, shelter, and love. We need to be respected in our community. We have a hunger for love, and for expressing our own being. All of these hungers, all of these needs, must be disciplined and controlled if society is to be successful."—**The Honorable Minister Louis Farrakhan**

(Ramadan: A Time for Healing, 2010)

Ramadan commemorates the revelation of the Holy Qur'an to Prophet Muhammad of Arabia (Peace Be Upon Him) some 1,400 years ago. Part of that revelation was a mandate that all Believers participate in a mental, spiritual, and physical fast. Muslims (and anyone else who desires to) must abstain from food, drink, and sexual intercourse during the daylight hours for a 30 day period. We are to focus on spiritual development, control anger, avoid arguments, make good habits, break bad habits, and read a portion of the Holy Qur'an daily.

Ramadan is a time to renew the spirit and re-establish discipline. Believers should strive to make all of their prayers, complete the reading of the entire Qur'an, abstain from unclean acts and thoughts, and engage in acts of kindness. Participation in the fast draws the Believer closer to Allah (God) by reminding him/her of the source of all his/her blessings.

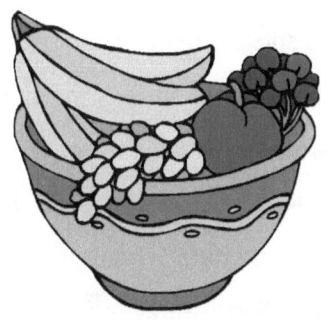

2 HOW TO EAT TO LIVE

"Eat a single meal a day, no matter what anyone says. If your doctor says that you should eat more than one meal, ignore him with a smile, and eat only once a day. If he tells you he eats three meals a day, tell him that his length of life is about the same as his patients. Then, tell the doctor to try eating one meal a day."—**The Honorable Elijah Muhammad** (Muhammad, 1967)

To ensure a long healthy life, eat one meal every 24-48 hours. That meal should consist of whole grains, navy beans, fruits, vegetables, whole milk, and healthy fats. The Messenger recommends a vegetarian lifestyle which consists of the best foods available. Consuming meat requires additional fluid consumption which can make staying hydrated a challenge during the fast. While certain fish and land animals are permitted, during Ramadan we are advised to abstain from their consumption. *How to Eat to Live* (Books 1 and 2) details which foods are best, which are permitted, foods that should be avoided, and foods that are forbidden. I will not delve into those specifics here; however, following the guidelines set out for us by the Most Honorable Elijah Muhammad will enable a successful Ramadan fast.

If you are following *How to Eat to Live,* making your Fajr prayers, and fasting at least three consecutive days every month, the transition into Ramadan will be less challenging. You will eat later than usual, maybe lose some sleep, and have to schedule reading/prayer time into your daily activities. Good planning will make for easy adjustments. Those who eat the wrong foods several times a day, fail to fast monthly, and skip the morning prayer will struggle to complete the fast and likely suffer symptoms of disease. All is not lost! If you follow the guidelines in Chapter 4 ("Preparing for the Fast"), you will improve your chances of reaping the full benefits of Ramadan.

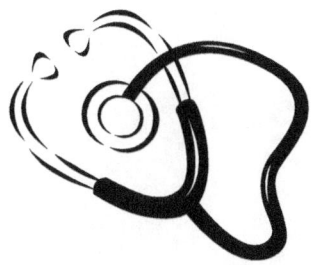

3 KNOW YOUR NUMBERS

Prior to the starting a fast, it is important to have a clear picture of your overall health condition. While fasting has many benefits, adults with diseases and chronic ailments like diabetes, high blood pressure, heart disease, and kidney disease, as well as those who take medications should consult their physicians for medical clearance. If you are ill, or completing a course of medication, your doctor may advise you to postpone the start of your fast. It is critical to obtain a detailed plan to manage your ailments if fasting is permitted.

Prior to the start of your fast, record your weight, waist measurement, and average number of hours of sleep per night. During the fast, weigh yourself and measure your waist once a week. Make dietary adjustments as needed. Pay close attention to the amount of sleep you get in relation to your energy levels, mood, and rate of perceived exertion. These numbers will provide you with a gauge of how well you manage your fast. Adjustments to your diet, exercise, hydration schedule, etc. will be more effective if you track your numbers.

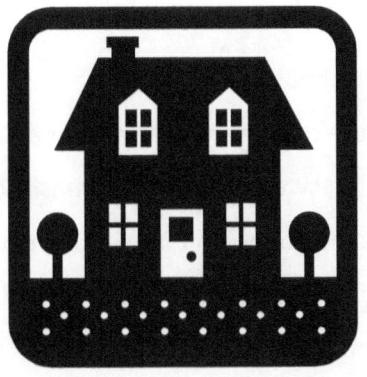

4 PREPARING FOR THE FAST

With success comes preparation. There are many things that can be done to ensure a successful fast. Here is my top ten list:

1. Eliminate unhealthy foods from your diet.
It is critical that we eat nutritionally-dense foods during Ramadan. Processed foods, fast food, junk food, etc. typically do not contain adequate amounts of protein and fiber. They also lack vitamins and minerals. You will still be hungry and want to eat more to compensate for the lack of nutritional value. You could potentially gain weight. Also, ensure that you eliminate bodily wastes regularly.

2. Reduce/eliminate caffeine intake.
Drinks that contain caffeine like coffee and green tea act as mild diuretics which will work against your efforts to stay hydrated. Make sure to get

adequate rest to conserve energy. Also, consuming slow-release carbohydrates will help keep your energy levels up.

3. Plan your meals and shop now.
Take inventory to ensure that you have sufficient amounts of healthy foods on hand. Consider: What will your diet consist of for the month? Will you eat salads, beans, soups, and fruit? How much time will you have to cook daily? Which foods can I cook in advance and freeze? Do I have enough water? Will I host iftar feasts?

4. Clean and organize your home.
Pay special attention to your kitchen and spaces where ablution, prayer, and reading will take place. Eliminate any clutter. Your home should be a restful and inviting refuge.

5. Take a moment to count your blessings.
Your attitude about Ramadan should be one of gratitude and humility. Be grateful for every blessing and trial. The way you start is the way you will end. If you focus on what you must sacrifice, you will miss out on the benefits.

6. Commit to making or breaking a habit.
Ramadan is a wonderful time to re-focus and establish discipline. If it takes 21 days to make or break a habit, then imagine where you will be in thirty!

7. Plan your day.

Your daily routine will require some adjustments. Be realistic about your limitations. You may decide to scale back non-essential tasks for the month. It may be necessary to change the time of day that you prepare meals. You may take naps before dinner. You may move your workouts to early morning so that you can drink. Choose the best time to complete your daily reading. Do what works for you.

8. See your doctor.

If possible, squeeze in a doctor's appointment. It is critical to know your numbers and how the fast may affect your overall health. The Ramadan fast can be quite beneficial for generally healthy people. If you are ill, pregnant, or breastfeeding, you should not be fasting. Those who take prescription medication due to existing health conditions may be unable to participate. Listen to your body and follow your doctor's orders.

9. Figure out the frequency and intensity of your workouts.

If you don't already follow an exercise regimen, this may not be the best time to start one. If you are currently active, adjust your workouts accordingly. You may work out 5-6 days and need to drop back to 3 or 4 days to conserve energy and manage hydration. Exercises like walking and yoga can help with circulation, mood, quality of sleep, and appetite control.

10. Adjust your daily schedule.

Start pushing dinner time later in the day. If you normally eat at 6pm, gradually delay your meal 15-20 minutes each day. Today, eat at 6:20 pm.

tomorrow, eat at 6:40 pm. Follow a similar regimen if you do not rise before dawn for prayer. Adjust your alarm clock 15 minutes earlier every day. By the start of the fast, your transition will be much easier.

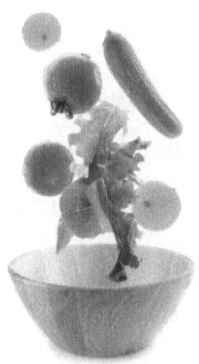

5 DIET AND NUTRITION

"The globally recogni(z)ed golden rule of dietary guidelines is that one should eat a variety of food using principles of moderation and balance. Usually, most health problems at this time are likely to arise from inappropriate diet or as a consequence of over-eating and insufficient sleep."

"Fasting also improves blood cholesterol profile, reduces gastric acidity, and prevents constipation and other digestive problems."

"Benefits of fasting appear only in those who maintain their diet, avoiding the high calorie and highly processed foods prepared during this time," -- Saijitha Sunil, Nutritionist/Dietician, Emirates Diagnostic Clinic (Zain, 2006)

Here are some very basic rules to follow that will ensure proper diet and nutrition during Ramadan:

1) Never allow your total daily caloric intake to drop below 1,200 calories
2) Prepare your own meals
3) Eat most of your vegetables cooked
4) Eat your fruits fresh (an hour before or after your meal)
5) Drink whole/raw milk daily
6) Drink a minimum of 64-96 ounces of water daily
7) Eat bean soup everyday
8) Eat whole wheat bread
9) Avoid desserts
10) Avoid fried foods
11) Avoid processed foods
12) Limit caffeine intake
13) Do not smoke
14) Do not consume alcohol
15) Take no drugs other than what is prescribed and necessary
16) Eat at the same time everyday

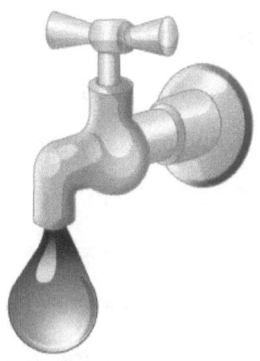

6 HYDRATION

The average individual requires 96 ounces (3 quarts) of water per day. For individuals who are participating in a weight loss program, an additional 8 ounce glass of water for every 25 pounds over ideal bodyweight is required. Extra hydration is also needed for those who live in warmer humid climates as well as those who perform brisk exercise. During Ramadan, the challenge lies in maintaining water intake levels within a shorter window of opportunity. In this chapter, we will cover the benefits of good hydration, how water is lost, causes of dehydration, effects of dehydration, hydration guidelines, foods to avoid, and foods to help stay hydrated during Ramadan.

There are many benefits to good hydration. The following systems and are positively affected: 1) endocrine gland function increases, 2) fluid retention is alleviated, 3) liver function improves which increases the percent of body fat percentage used for energy (which promotes weight loss), 4) natural thirst returns, 5) appetite decreases significantly, 6) metabolic functions improve, 7) nutrients are well distributed throughout the body, 8) body temperature regulation improves, and 9) blood volume is maintained. (Micheal A. Clark, 2008)

The human body loses water daily through a variety of methods. It is excreted as urine (1500 mL), eliminated in the feces (200 mL), lost in expired breath (300 mL), secreted as sweat by a resting adult at ambient air temperature of 68 degrees Fahrenheit (100 mL), and lost as cutaneous transpiration that diffuses through the epidermis and evaporates (400 mL). Humid weather and prolonged heavy work causes increases in perspiration and respiratory water loss from 650 mL up to 5L per day. (Saladin, 2007)

Dehydration is caused by any of the following: 1) below minimum fluid intake, 2) exercise in hot/humid climates, 3) consuming beverages high in caffeine, 4) excessive protein intake, 5) alcohol consumption, 6) consuming excess sodium, 7) use of laxatives/diuretics, 8) prolonged physical activity without fluid replacement. (Heather Hedrick Fink, 2009)

Failure to maintain proper hydration has many adverse effects on the human body. Dehydration causes any or all of the following: 1) decreased blood volume, 2) increased heart rate, 3) decreased performance, 4) sodium retention, 5) decreased blood pressure, 6) decreased cardiac output, 7) decreased sweat rate, 8) decreased blood flow to skin, 9) increased core temperature, 10) increased perceived exertion, 11) water retention, and 12) increased use of muscle glycogen. (Micheal A. Clark, 2008)

To monitor hydration levels, here are some guidelines to follow:

- ✓ Check urine to ensure a pale yellow color. The darker your urine is, the more dehydrated you are.
- ✓ Consume foods and beverages that have high water content.
- ✓ Avoid caffeine in any form.
- ✓ Eliminate alcohol consumption.
- ✓ Eat a balanced diet including moderate amounts of protein.
- ✓ Be aware of diuretic side effects of medications. Consult your doctor.
- ✓ Exercise in cooler temperatures during periods when you can drink.
- ✓ Drink enough water to replace water lost during exercise. For every pound lost, drink 16-24 ounces of water. Another option is to drink 7-10 ounces for every 10-20 minutes of exercise.

(Heather Hedrick Fink, 2009)

Foods that should be avoided during the fast include caffeine, green tea, protein in excess of daily requirements, excess sodium, alcohol, diuretics, laxatives beyond occasional use, sodas.

Foods that will help keep you hydrated include fruits, vegetables, water, raw milk, soups, fresh juices, smoothies, and shakes. Being able to drink beverages with high vitamin and mineral content is a plus.

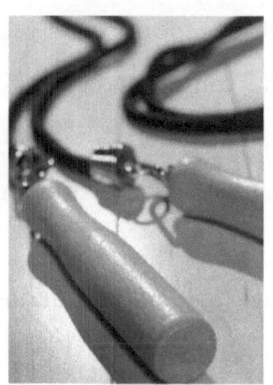

7 EXERCISE AND WEIGHT MANAGEMENT

"Continuing to exercise is a healthy way to enjoy Ramadan. It maintains mizan or balance. Balance is achieved when the spiritual, mental, and physical life is maintained.

"During Ramadan the spirit is kept healthy by purging the self of all negativity, including the negativity that may be associated with the fast. The mental self is maintained through regular reading of the Quran. The physical self is kept strong through a light workout." (Green, 2009)

It is important to treat your body well during Ramadan. Active people will have to pay particularly close attention to nutrition, hydration levels, and quality of sleep/rest. Many see Ramadan as an opportunity to lose weight. If you are not currently participating in an exercise program, Ramadan is not the time to start strenuous workouts. Moderate physical activity is recommended.

If you eliminate bad foods from your diet, eat balanced meals, stay hydrated, control your portions, stay active (without over-exerting yourself), and rest when needed, your body will become more efficient at metabolizing your food, utilizing fat for energy, releasing excess fluid and toxins, and ultimately lose some unwanted pounds.

Your health and fitness goals during Ramadan should be realistic. The positive effects of the fast should be a great starting place for living a healthier lifestyle. Reverting back to old habits after Ramadan ends is counter-productive and may be more harmful to your body than not taking the fast at all.

Those who exercise regularly should consider performing their workouts before the sun rises or after the sun sets when they can drink. In addition to the required water intake for the day, exercisers should drink during the workout to replace water lost through sweat, metabolic processes, and exerting themselves. It may be necessary to split a hard workout up into two parts (performing one part early and the other late in the day). Some may opt to performing intense exercises for shorter durations on alternate days. Reducing the number of days altogether during the fasting period may be more desirable. Lifting lighter weights with higher repetitions is a good way to preserve muscle mass without over-exertion. The key is to have clearly defined fitness goals, create a plan to achieve them, and pay attention to how your body responds.

For those who do not exercise regularly, walking everyday for at least 20 minutes early in the morning is a good baseline goal. Light toning and stretching exercises are beneficial as well. Staying active will help avoid constipation, aid in digestion, maintain/improve metabolism, and aid in elimination of toxins.

8 PROPER REST

The amount and quality of sleep one experiences affects endocrine system function, mood, energy levels, and recovery of all major systems. During Ramadan, sleep quantity and quality can be affected by late meals, the need to rise early for prayer and breakfast, caffeine intake (due to its stimulant and diuretic effects), and the reduced number of uninterrupted hours of sleep. Hyper-hydration will also lead to frequent urination which also interrupts one's rest.

Managing proper rest can take many forms. Several nutritional and therapeutic factors have been identified as sleep enhancers including: melatonin, tryptophan, valerian root and other sedative herbs, consuming a high Glycemic Index meal prior to bedtime, warming the skin, hydrotherapy, following a sleep hygiene regimen, and maintaining a balanced, healthy diet.

To compensate for lost sleep, it is recommended that naps lasting less than 45 minutes in duration be taken early in the day. Elevate your feet whenever possible. Maintain moderate physical activity and manage stress levels. Also, avoid falling asleep in front of the television. (Halson, 2008)

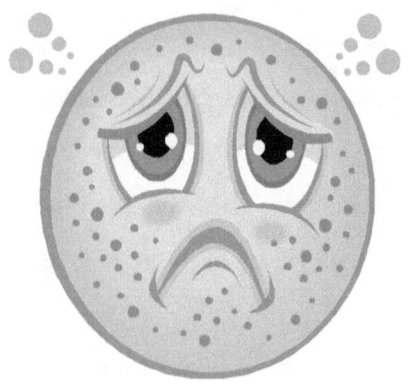

9 SIDE EFFECTS OF FASTING

Fasting may present some side effects. Those who take the fast have reported headaches, dizziness, acne, flu-like symptoms, and fatigue. These symptoms are often attributed to detoxification. Toxins are stored in body fat. If fat is used for fuel during the day, these toxins are released into the bloodstream. Without fluid consumption, these toxins are slower to exit the body thus causing discomfort. Other health risks include: heartburn, poor control of diabetes, dehydration, constipation, stress and weight control. In this chapter, we will cover ways to alleviate these symptoms. Remember, listen to your body and follow your doctor's orders. It is better to make up a like number of days rather to risk your health.

Upon rising in the morning, squeeze the juice of a lemon into your water. The vitamin C will give your immune system a boost and help fight off disease. The acid from the lemon will reduce intestinal parasites which can cause some gastrointestinal distress. Be sure to ingest up to half of your required fluid intake for the day before sunrise. Hydration, proper diet, and adequate rest will help keep headaches at bay. Persistent flu-like symptoms, headaches, and dizziness should be reported to your physician. Additional rest may be needed during the day. The key is to listen to your body and give it what it needs. A little pampering goes a long way.

Heartburn is a common issue during the fast. While fasting normally reduces the amount of stomach acid produced for digestion and killing bacteria, seeing, smelling, and even thinking about food may signal the stomach to produce more acid. The result is gastrointestinal discomfort including heartburn. Eliminating fried and spicy foods along with caffeine and smoking are recommended to alleviate symptoms. Sleeping with the head elevated on a pillow can also bring relief. (Fasting: Health Risks)

Diabetics who rely on insulin injections to control blood sugar levels should not participate in the Ramadan fast. Those who use oral medication and/or diet to manage the disease should consult their physicians prior to the starting the fast. It is critical that patients follow their doctor's orders and react quickly to adverse symptoms, even if it means breaking the fast. Diabetics who exercise should adjust their workout schedules accordingly. They should discuss with their care providers if taking the fast is feasible, how to manage meals and medications, specific diet recommendations, and timing, frequency, and intensity of exercise. Regular glucose testing is essential:

"Regular self-monitoring of your blood glucose is strongly advised. Low blood sugar levels (a 'hypo') are dangerous, and if untreated may lead to fainting or fits.

"Feeling dizzy, sweaty and disoriented may all suggest a hypo. If a person with diabetes has these symptoms, they should immediately have a sugary drink, or place sugar or a sugar-rich sweet below their tongue." (Fasting: Health Risks)

Dehydration is one of the most common conditions that develops during Ramadan. The causes range from inadequate fluid intake to prolonged physical activity without hydration. Chapter 6 of this book ("Hydration") details the causes of dehydration and how to avoid it. In the event that dehydration does occur, be prepared to break your fast. Dizziness, becoming disoriented, and fainting require immediate hydration and, potentially, medical attention. Consult your physician prior to resuming the fast.

Constipation can be avoided by drinking plenty of water, whole milk, and fresh juices while consuming foods that contain high amounts of fiber and water. Examples include, but are not limited to, fruits, vegetables, beans, soups, and whole grains. Physical activities like walking and light exercise are also recommended. Taking additional fiber or an herbal laxative may bring short-term relief. (Fasting: Health Risks)

Without adequate preparation, Ramadan can be stressful. Participants may struggle with rising earlier than usual. Eating at different times of the day, working, family obligations, making the required prayers, food preparation, school, being unable to drink, managing health, inadequate rest, and more can take the focus away from the purpose and intention of the fast. It is important to be realistic about what this 30 day period will look like for YOU. Do not over-commit yourself. Know your limits. Avoid negative people and situations. Control your anger. Eat well and drink sufficiently. Pray. Pray. Pray. During this month, take a break from television, the computer, and social media beyond essential tasks. Scale back your workouts: focus on quality versus quantity. Keep your home clutter-free.

Body weight has been known to fluctuate during Ramadan. Initially, many experience a loss in the form of water weight. This can be a result of reduced fluid intake. One of the benefits of the fast is that the digestive system gets a break. The remaining systems can efficiently utilize food for fuel, tissue growth, and tissue repair. Circulation improves and excess fluid build-up is excreted from the body as waste. Loss of appetite may make it difficult to maintain normal calorie intake. Hydration curbs appetite, so when breaking the fast it is critical to consume juicy fruits, vegetables, and soups to satisfy both caloric and hydration needs. To avoid unwanted weight gain, it is critical to eat nutritionally-dense foods. Monitor portion-sizes, consume fresh fruits and vegetables, avoid excessive sugar and salt, avoid processed foods, drink plenty of water, consume navy beans, lentils, and raw milk, and choose healthy whole grains. Lastly, it is important to maintain a consistent level of physical activity. Doing so will encourage use of body fat to fuel movement and metabolic processes. (Refer to Chapter 7.)

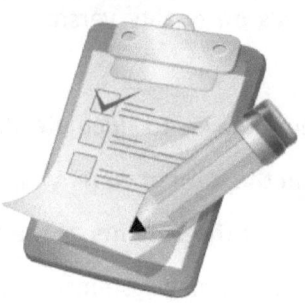

10 YOUR RAMADAN PLAN

Putting together your Ramadan strategy takes simple planning and preparation. Here is a recap of things to consider:

1) Clean up your diet and adjust your eating time and frequency.
2) Consult your doctor to ensure good health prior to the fast.
3) Prepare your home by cleaning and de-cluttering.
4) Plan meals and shop to ensure adequate supplies.
5) Adjust sleep patterns.
6) Review monthly schedule and limit activities to essential tasks.
7) Make a plan for exercise.
8) Make plans to accommodate prayer.
9) Create a strategy for make-up days.

10) Focus on the benefits of Ramadan and be grateful for your
blessings!

Ramadan Mubarak!

BIBLIOGRAPHY

Fasting: Health Risks. 26 July 2011
<http://www.nhs.uk/Livewell/Healthyramadan/Pages/fastinghealthris
ks.aspx>.

Green, Khalil. Islam at Suite 101. 13 August 2009. 28 July 2011
<http://www.suite101.com/content/staying-fit-during-ramadan-
a139013>.

Halson, Shona L. "Nutrition, Sleep, and Recovery." European Journal of
Sport Science (2008): 119-126.

Heather Hedrick Fink, Lisa A. Burgoon, Alan E. Mikesky. Practical
Applications in Sports Nutrition. 2nd Edition. Jones and Bartlett
Publishers, LLC, 2009.

Micheal A. Clark, Scott Lucett, Rodney J. Corn. NASM Essentials of
Personal Fitness Training, 3rd ed. Lippincott, Williams, and Wilkins,
2008.

Muhammad, Elijah. "How to Eat to Live, Book One." Chicago:
Muhammad's Temple of Islam No. 2, 1967. 9.

Ramadan: A Time for Healing. 10 August 2010. 26 July 2011
<http://www.finalcall.com/artman/publish/Perspectives_1/article_71
91.shtml>.

Saladin, Kenneth S. Anatomy and Physiology: The Unity of Form and
Function. 4th Edition. New York: McGraw Hill Companies, 2007.

Zain, Asma Ali. Eat the Right Food During Ramadan. 24 September
2006. 26 July 2011
<http://www.khaleejtimes.com/DisplayArticleNew.asp?xfile=data/the
uae/2006/September/theuae_September805.xml&section=theuae&c
ol>.

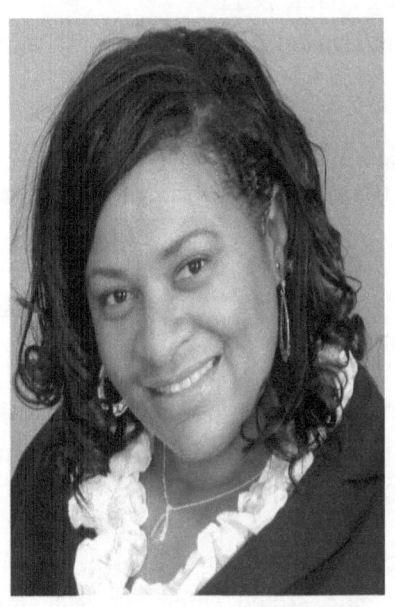

ABOUT THE AUTHOR

Raychelle Muhammad holds a B.S. in Sports Management. She is also certified as a personal trainer by the National Academy of Sports Medicine. Raychelle is a published author and illustrator of children's and family books. Her blog (http://www.journeysfit.blogspot.com) covers a wide range of health and wellness topics. Raychelle enjoys urban gardening, interior design, and cooking. She is married and has one daughter whom she homeschools.

www.ingramcontent.com/pod-product-compliance
Lightning Source LLC
Chambersburg PA
CBHW061233280526
45784CB00006B/2745